Activities for the Family Caregiver

PARKINSON'S DISEASE

R.O.S.

HOW TO ENGAGE
HOW TO LIVE

Scott Silknitter
Robert D. Brennan, RN, NHA, MS, CDP
Dawn Worsley, ADC/MC/EDU, CDP

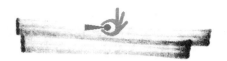

Disclaimer

This book is for informational purposes only and is not intended as medical advice, diagnosis, or treatment. Always seek advice from a qualified physician about medical concerns, and do not disregard medical advice because of something you read in this book. This book does not replace the need for diagnostic evaluation, ongoing physician care, and professional assessment of treatments. Every effort has been made to make this book as complete and helpful as possible. It is important, however, for this book to be used as a resource and idea-generating guide and not as an ultimate source for a plan of care.

ISBN # 978-1518611162

Published by
R.O.S. Therapy Systems, L.L.C.
Greensboro, NC
888-352-9788
www.ROSTherapySystems.com

Activities for the Family Caregiver— Parkinson's Disease

This book is a general guide for family caregivers covering the basics of Activities and Activities of Daily Living for someone with Parkinson's disease. It is based on the principles and approaches used in the training and certification of long-term care professionals. This book incorporates common sense and practical information for things like engaging, bathing, and feeding your loved one. It is part of the R.O.S. Activities for the Family Caregiver book series, which is designed to help caregivers engage the ones for whom they care.

With the assistance of industry-leading professionals, we have written this book for you in the hopes of providing helpful "How To's" for engaging with your loved one.

Of all the books in our Activities for the Family Caregiver series, this book and the *Activities 101 for the Family Caregiver—Parkinson's Disease* have a special meaning for me. Our company began as a simple backyard project specifically to help my mother and father in my dad's 25-year battle with Parkinson's and dementia.

Please have other family members and caregivers of your loved one read this book as well. Use this as a tool to break down the walls of isolation for you and your loved one. Make sure everyone is on the same page.

From our family of caregivers to yours, please remember that you are not alone, and to never give up.

Scott Silknitter

Family Members and Caregivers
that have read this book:

_____

_____

_____

_____

_____

_____

_____

_____

_____

_____

_____

_____

Table of Contents

Chapter 1

Parkinson's Disease Overview

Parkinson's disease affects the way you move. It happens when there is a problem with certain nerve cells in the brain.

Normally, these nerve cells make a chemical called dopamine that sends signals to the part of your brain that controls movement. Dopamine lets your muscles move smoothly and do what you want them to do. When you have Parkinson's, these nerve cells break down, your body's dopamine production slows, and you have trouble moving the way you want to move.

Parkinson's is progressive, meaning it gets worse over time, and it affects every individual differently. The progression can happen slowly over many years or faster in a shorter period of time. Initially there will be small changes in your loved one, but they will be able to function fairly independently. As the disease progresses, they will need more and more assistance. As a caregiver, you will see firsthand what is happening, how it affects your loved one, and what needs to be done. You must help your loved one adjust accordingly.

Below is an adaptation from the Family Caregiver Alliance® of the Hoehn and Yahr scale which gives a good overview of the stages of Parkinson's that caregivers must be aware of in order to adjust the assistance to be given and activities to be planned for their loved one.

Family Caregiver Alliance® Adaptation of Hoehn and Yahr Scale

Symptoms Prior to Diagnosis

Symptoms include depression, anxiety, fatigue, disturbance of color vision, constipation, loss of smell acuity, problems with sleep, and slowed thinking.

Stage 1

Motor symptoms develop on one side
of the body.

Stage 2

Symptoms spread to both sides of the body.

Stage 3

Balance starts to become impaired.

Stage 4

More difficulty develops with gait, freezing or
small, fast steps.

More problems that affect the center or
midline of the body develop, e.g., difficulty
with swallowing and balance, and increased
nonmotor problems.

Stage 5

Inability to locomote independently results
in dependency on a wheelchair or other
mobility device.

Patience is a virtue. As the primary caregiver, your patience will be tested, especially if you are tired or are in a stressful situation. With the progression of the disease, your loved one may need more time to accomplish tasks. Be patient and give your loved one the opportunity to be successful no matter the task. Make sure that all caregivers for your loved one understand that as well. There will be a point when caregivers have to step in and assist in almost every task, but until that happens, give your loved one a chance to be successful and maintain self-confidence.

As the primary family caregiver—husband, wife, son, or daughter—your relationship and role with your loved one will change along with the progression of the disease. You will become the cheerleader, motivator, protector, activity director, social coordinator, nurse, and maybe even parent to your loved one. You must prepare yourself for this role as much as possible.

With activities based on <u>personal preference and ability</u>, people with Parkinson's can still live a full life. One of the keys to living a full life is to engage in active activities such as walking, dancing, gardening, tai chi, yoga, or even folding laundry to keep the body active. It is also important to engage in mindful, creative, and social activities, such as playing cards, working crossword puzzles, playing checkers, talking with friends, painting, listening to music, or playing trivia games, to keep the mind and parts of the body active. Use it or lose it, as the saying goes.

There are four main symptoms of Parkinson's. You and your loved one may initially notice just one. The symptoms are:

1. Tremor, which means shaking or trembling. Tremor may affect your hands, arms or legs.
2. Stiff muscles.
3. Slow movement.
4. Problems with balance or walking.

Again, Parkinson's disease affects each individual differently. For example, many people experience a tremor, while others might not have tremors, but might have problems with balance.

In time, Parkinson's will affect muscles throughout your loved one's body. As this happens, you will need to adjust the time necessary or the tools used to allow your loved one to participate in an activity.

As the primary family caregiver, you need to know and understand the various symptoms of Parkinson's so that you can adjust schedules, levels of participation, and the time it takes to participate accordingly. You will also need to educate family, friends, and other caregivers about what your loved one may be experiencing and why. The following pages provide basic descriptions of Parkinson's symptoms that may affect your loved one.

Primary Symptoms
of Parkinson's Disease

Resting Tremor

Although this is the most noticeable sign of the disease, not all people with Parkinson's will develop a tremor.

As an example, there may be a tremor in one finger. The tremor, a shaking or trembling movement, usually appears when your loved one's muscles are at rest or relaxed, thus the term "resting tremor." The finger or other affected body part trembles when it is not performing an action.

The tremor usually stops when a person begins an action.

The tremor can spread to the other side of the body as the disease progresses, but usually remains most apparent on the side initially affected. Please note that the Parkinson's tremor can be intensified by stress or excitement.

A tremor may attract what you or your loved one perceives to be unwanted attention. If it is noticed, use it as a teachable moment to educate others about Parkinson's. Do not be ashamed or embarrassed about Parkinson's disease. It is a part of who your loved one is.

Stiff Muscles or Rigidity

Muscles normally stretch when they move and then relax when they are at rest. Rigidity causes stiffness and inflexibility of the limbs, neck, and trunk.

Rigidity in Parkinson's disease means the muscle of your loved one's affected limb is always stiff and does not relax. This can contribute to a decreased range of motion.

One of the more common symptoms that your loved one may experience is tightness of the neck, shoulder, and/or leg. Rigidity can be uncomfortable or even painful.

Here are some examples of the challenges your loved one may experience as a result of their stiff or rigid muscles:

- A challenge getting in and out of the car for an outing to the store, a doctor's appointment, or a trip to the park.

- A challenge enjoying activities such as dancing, taking a walk, turning their head to see an event or speak with someone who is not facing them directly.

- A challenge performing tasks such as potting plants, holding playing cards, sorting coins, or grasping and placing puzzle pieces.

- A challenge getting in or out of a chair or bed.

Slow Movement or Bradykinesia

Slow movement or bradykinesia describes a general reduction of spontaneous movement.

It can give the appearance of stillness or a decrease in facial expressivity, and it can make it difficult to perform repetitive movements.

With bradykinesia, your loved one may walk with short, shuffling steps. Your loved one with both rigidity and bradykinesia might not swing their arms when walking.

In addition, your loved one's speech may be affected. It may become quieter and less distinct as the disease progresses due to the reduction and limited range of movement caused by bradykinesia.

Here are some examples of the challenges your loved one may experience as a result of slow movement or bradykinesia:

- A challenge with activities of daily living such as buttoning a shirt, cutting food, or brushing teeth.

- A challenge having a conversation or answering questions in a timeframe that meets someone else's expectation of the appropriate length of time. As the caregiver, you must ensure that others give your loved one time to speak.

- A challenge with repetitive movements such as writing, tapping a finger, moving a foot to the rhythm of music, or dialing a phone number.

Problems with Balance/Walking, or Postural Instability

Problems with balance/walking, or postural instability, is another symptom of Parkinson's disease. Postural instability is a tendency to be unstable when standing upright. With postural instability, your loved one has lost some of the reflexes needed for maintaining an upright posture. This means your loved one could fall backwards. They may also have difficulty making turns or quick movements.

Retropulsion means your loved one may have a tendency to sway backwards when rising from a chair, standing or turning. It can result in a backward fall.

Examples of how problems with balance/walking or postural instability can affect being active or engaging in activities:

- A challenge getting up from a chair unassisted in order to move from one room to another.

- A challenge taking a walk.

- A challenge standing for pictures with family or friends.

- A challenge dancing with a loved one.

- A challenge with outdoor activities such as gardening.

Secondary Symptoms
of Parkinson's Disease

In addition to the primary symptoms of Parkinson's, there are other secondary motor symptoms your loved one may experience.

Freezing

Gait is defined as a person's manner of walking, stepping or running. People who experience freezing will normally hesitate before stepping forward. They feel like their feet are glued to the floor. Freezing is often temporary, and a person can enter a normal stride once he or she gets past the first step.

Freezing can occur in very specific situations, such as when a person is starting to walk, pivoting, crossing a threshold or doorway, and when approaching a chair.

Some individuals have severe freezing, in which they simply cannot take a step. Freezing is a potentially serious problem in Parkinson's disease, as it may increase a person's risk of falling forward. Various types of cues, such as an exaggerated first step, can help with freezing.

Mask-like Expression

A person with Parkinson's may develop what is referred to as a mask-like expression or face, where the muscles in the face "freeze" into a mask-like or serious expression. Unable to show happiness with a simple smile or sadness with a frown, the mask of Parkinson's can seriously impact your loved one's ability to convey genuine emotions, and can affect your ability to read your loved one's nonverbal communication cues.

Unwanted Accelerations

Some people with Parkinson's experience movement or speech that is involuntarily quick or hurried. People with fast speech may produce a rapid stammering that is hard to understand.

Others may experience festination, which is an uncontrollable acceleration in gait that may increase the risk for falls.

Additional secondary motor symptoms that your loved one may experience and that can affect your loved one's ability to enjoy an activity or to be active include the following:

- Stooped posture and a tendency to lean forward

- Difficulty swallowing

- Sexual dysfunction

- Cramping

- Drooling

- Speech problems, such as softness of voice or slurred speech caused by lack of muscle control.

Nonmotor Symptoms

In addition to the motor symptoms, most people with Parkinson's disease will experience nonmotor symptoms that can affect their ability to fully participate in an activity or be active. Nonmotor symptoms are those that do not involve movement, coordination, physical tasks or mobility. While a person's family and friends might not be able to see them, these symptoms might be more challenging for your loved one than the motor impairments. As the caregiver, you need to be a detective to discover and identify these symptoms to minimize as best as possible their impact on your loved one's ability to engage in an activity. Nonmotor symptoms of Parkinson's include:

- Loss of sense of smell

- Mood disorders

- Sleep disturbances

- Constipation

- Bladder problems

- Excessive saliva

- Weight loss or gain

- Vision and dental problems

- Soft speech

- Fatigue and loss of energy

- Depression

- Fear and anxiety

- Skin problems

- Cognitive issues, such as memory difficulties, slowed thinking, confusion, and in some cases, dementia.

Parkinson's Disease and Dementia

In simple terms, dementia is a loss of brain function that can affect memory, thinking, language, judgment, and behavior. Some common symptoms of dementia include:

- Memory loss

- Impaired judgment and difficulties with thinking

- Loss of communication skills

- Inappropriate behavior

- Disorientation as to time and place

- Gait, motor, and balance problems

- Neglect of personal care and safety

- Hallucinations, paranoia, and agitation

When combined with the symptoms of Parkinson's, these can make life very stressful.

Consider the following set of circumstances: Your loved one has a neurologist appointment. Your loved one does not remember that they have an appointment, they do not recognize the front of the office building from the parking lot, and they do not recognize you. They think you are there to drop them off and leave them forever. Their legs are stiff, and they cannot easily get out of the car. The stress of not understanding causes their entire body to freeze when they are finally able to get out of the car.

This is a challenge that you did not expect, but must plan for. It is an instance where your planning, patience, communication skills, and flexibility will be tested.

Planning, patience, effective communication, and the ability to adapt are all easier said than done if you are in the heat of the moment where everything that could happen, does happen. Please remember that your loved one did not choose to be in this situation, and that the effects of Parkinson's are as frustrating for your loved one as they are for you. If they could choose not to have Parkinson's and/or dementia, they would not have it. As the disease progresses, you might not know what the day is going to hold or even if it will be a good day or a bad day. You must use all of the resources available to you, such as this book, to be ready when something unexpected and/or unplanned does happen. Accept help when it is offered, and take time to take care of yourself whenever the opportunity arises. As much as it may feel like it at certain times, you are not alone in this fight.

Chapter 2

Activities, Their Benefits, and the Family

"Activities" and "Activities of Daily Living" (ADLs) are critical aspects to caring for a loved one at home. Both leisure and daily living activities require knowledge of your loved one's habits, preferences, abilities, and routines. Caregivers need to have the ability to communicate with and execute a planned activity with your loved one. Life happens, and things can happen spontaneously, but all activities should be planned to offer the best possible outcome to enhance your loved one's sense of well-being. Activities should promote or enhance your loved one's physical, cognitive, and emotional health. In this book, we will focus on leisure activities and the activities of daily living with common sense suggestions and tips on the "How To's" of getting your loved one engaged, dressed, and fed.

In the institutional setting of today, leisure activities are required by law if a nursing home accepts government funding. In these situations, activities are to be provided to every resident on a daily basis based on an individual's preferences. Activities has grown into a profession where Certified Activity Professionals and their staff plan and execute activity programs for residents and seniors in their care. It is NOT just bingo.

In addition, staff members are required to undergo annual training on the basics of Activities of Daily Living in order to provide better care for the residents they work with.

This book was made for the millions of families and informal caregivers who care for their loved ones with Parkinson's disease at home. Recognizing the growth in the numbers of those aging in place due to financial need or desire to just be at home, the R.O.S. Activities 101/201 Programs and this book are based on the principles and approaches used by professionals in skilled settings. This was done for two reasons.

1. Provide family caregivers the knowledge and tools to allow them to engage their loved one so that both can enjoy the benefits of activities.
2. Offer a starting point that will provide continuity of approach regarding care, communication, and information-gathering to minimize changes and acclimation time if your loved one does have to move from home to an institutional setting.

If you choose to use the services of a home care agency while caring for your loved one at home, please ask if they have a Home Care Certified professional on staff, and make sure that the caregiver you choose has received basic training on Leisure Activities and Activities of Daily Living. This will assist with continuity of approach, communication, and planning that will benefit both you and your loved one.

Our goal is to help you deliver meaningful programs of interest to your loved one that focus on physical, social, spiritual, cognitive, and recreational activities. Everyone involved in the care for your loved one should be "on the same page" to minimize changes and challenges that your loved one will face.

Not all family members may understand or accept your loved one's Parkinson's disease. Your loved one may look the same on the outside and may be having a "good day" when someone comes to visit. Family members who visit occasionally might not understand or see all of the symptoms that primary caregivers see daily. They may underestimate or minimize the responsibilities or stress. This can create conflict. If it helps to avoid a conflict or stress, please have the family members read this book prior to a visit so they can begin to understand the monumental task that you face as a caregiver. Use visits and interactions as teaching moments.

The Benefits of Activities
with a Standard Approach

Caregiver Benefits of Standard Approach to Activities

Planned and well-executed activities result in less stress for the caregiver as well as less stress for your loved one. Whether it is playing a game or bathing, a standard approach where as many details are planned as possible, can make a significant, positive difference for everyone.

Social Benefits of Activities

Activities offer the opportunity for increased social interaction between family members, friends, caregivers, and the one being cared for. Activities create positive experiences and memories for everyone.

Behavioral Benefits of Activities

Well-planned and well-executed activities of any type can reduce challenging behaviors that sometimes arise when caring for someone with Parkinson's disease.

Self-Esteem Benefits of Activities

Leisure activities offered at the right skill level provide your loved one with an opportunity for success. This is also true with activities of daily living such as dressing. Success during activities improves how your loved one feels about themselves.

Sleep Benefits of Activities

When they are regularly incorporated into a daily routine, activities can improve sleeping at night. If a loved one is inactive all day, it is likely they will nap periodically. Napping can interrupt good sleep patterns at night.

Being a primary caregiver is a 24/7 job. Without help, you are always on call and run the risk of becoming physically and mentally exhausted.

When you do bring in help, make sure all of your loved one's caregivers (full-time, part-time, family, and friends) use the same approach for activities and interaction that you do. With a common approach, there are significantly less opportunities to disrupt routines and make unsettling changes that affect you and your loved one long after the help has left.

A common approach is key. Demand it!

The Four Pillars of Activities

The R.O.S. Activities 101/201 Programs focus on the Four Pillars of Activities. These are areas that all caregivers for your loved one should be familiar with to provide continuity of care and give your loved one the greatest opportunity for success to engage and improve the quality of life for everyone.

First Pillar of Activities: Know your Loved One—Information Gathering and Assessment

Have a Personal History Form completed. Know them—who they are, who they were, and what their functional abilities are today. Make sure all caregivers know this as well.

Second Pillar of Activities: Communicating and Motivating for Success

Communication is key. Each caregiver must know how to effectively communicate with your loved one and be consistent with techniques.

Third Pillar of Activities: Customary Routines and Preferences

As best as possible, maintain a routine and daily plan based on your loved one's needs and preferences.

Fourth Pillar of Activities: Planning and Executing Activities

Based on all of the information you have gathered about your loved one, you have the opportunity to offer engaging activities that are appropriate and meet your loved one's personal preferences.

Chapter 3

First Pillar of Activities:
Know Your Loved One—
Information Gathering
and Assessment

Before you begin providing personal care, you need to recognize various personal attributes and abilities of your loved one and yourself. The more you know about your loved one's lifestyle, likes, and dislikes, the easier providing for their personal and leisure needs will be.

It is important to concentrate on what your loved one **CAN DO**, not what they **CANNOT DO**. The more you know about your loved one, the more effective you can be as a caregiver to them. Caregiving routines should be kept structured and regular.

Knowing your loved one's individual needs, interests, functional abilities, and capacities will assist you in knowing how to plan and engage in meaningful and quality leisure activities. This is the First Pillar of Activities and will help in designing activities that your loved one can enjoy.

As the primary caregiver, you may already know most of the answers to the items listed below, but recording them in a Personal History Form is a good and necessary exercise for you, other family members, and other caregivers to complete. The following are items about your loved one that you are most likely able to provide yourself:

Basic Information
Name, preferred name to be called, age, and date of birth

Background Information
Place of birth, cultural/ethnic background, marital status, children (how many, and their names), religion/church, military

service/employment, education level, and primary language spoken

Medical and Dietary/Nutritional Information

Any formal diagnosis, allergies, and food regimen/diets

Habits

Drinking/alcohol, smoking, exercise, and other things that are a daily habit

Physical Status

Abilities/limitations, visual aids, hearing deficits, speech, communication, hand dominance, and mobility/gait

Mental Status

Alertness, cognitive abilities/limitations, orientation to family, time, place, person, routine, etc.

Social Status

One-on-one interaction, being visited, communication with others through written words, phone calls or other means

Emotional Status

Level of contentment, outgoing/withdrawn, extroverted/introverted, dependent/independent

Leisure Status

Past, present, and possible future interests

Vision Status

Any visual impairment they may have.

Informal Assessments

To complement the information that you yourself can provide about your loved one, you will want to include additional information from other sources. We use the term "informal assessments" to describe interviews with family members and others who regularly interact with your loved one, as well as observations and information gathered through other means.

Interviews

The interview process is particularly important for someone who is experiencing some of the effects of Parkinson's that make communication difficult, such as slowed or slurred speech, or a mask-like expression. These can easily lead to a person avoiding personal interaction and becoming socially isolated. Help your loved one and others break through these barriers by gathering as much information as possible and sharing it with all caregivers—family, informal, and formal. Interviews can be done in person, over the phone, or by asking someone to fill out the Personal History Form as much as they can.

Observations

Observations are what you and others have seen or heard concerning your loved one. How do they interact with others? What have you observed about your loved one's behavior? How does your loved one respond to questions or statements made by others?

What kind of body language and expressions do they use to express their feelings? You have probably seen these interactions a thousand times and made a mental note whenever something stuck out. Now, you must write them down for your future use and for others.

Information Gathered Through Other Means

Make a request of family members or friends to help complete a Personal History Form for your loved one. An example of this form is located at the end of this section.

Your ability to identify past preferences is vital to the planning and execution of an activity, which we will cover in this book.

Details matter. Let's look at someone who enjoys gardening.

During their assessments, four people might all say they like "gardening," yet they might not actually have the same activity in mind or enjoy the same activity.

- Person 1—Enjoys going outside, cutting the grass, trimming the hedges, and weed whacking. Anything less would not meet his preference.

- Person 2—Enjoys getting in the flower beds, planting flowers and vegetables, and tending to her garden on her hands and knees each day for an hour.

- Person 3—Enjoys indoor plants, propagating plants, and watering and caring for plants daily.

- Person 4—Enjoys arranging flowers in vases for tables.

As you can see from these examples, details matter. Gather as much information as you can for yourself and all family members and caregivers who may help with your loved one.

The R.O.S. Personal History Form is a starting point to gather as much information as possible. You may download a copy of the Personal History Form at www.ROSTherapySystems.com.

Personal History Form

This is _____'s Personal History

Name: _____

Maiden Name: _____

Date of Birth: _____

Preferred Name: _____

Name and relationship of people completing this history:

_____

_____

_____

What age do you think the person thinks they are?

_____

Do they ask for their spouse but do not recognize them?

_____

Do they look for their children but do not recognize them?

_____

Do they look for their mom? _____

Do they perceive themselves as younger? Please describe.

_____

_____

_____

Describe the "home" they remember. _____

_____

_____

_____

Describe the person's personality prior to the onset of the
disease._____

_____

_____

What makes the person feel valued? Talents, occupation,
accomplishments, family, etc. _____

_____

_____

What are some favorite items they must always have in
sight or close by? _____

_____

_____

What is their exact morning routine? _____

_____

_____

_____

What is their exact evening routine? _____

_____

_____

_____

_____

What type of clothing do they prefer? Do they like to choose their own clothes for the day or do they prefer to have their clothes laid out for them?

_____

_____

_____

_____

What is their favorite beverage?

_____

What is their favorite food?

_____

What will get them motivated? (Church, friends coming over, going out, etc.)

_____

_____

_____

_____

List significant interests in their life, such as hobbies, recreational activities, job related skills/experiences, military experience, etc.

- Age 8 to 20:

_____

_____

_____

- Age 20 to 40:

_____

_____

_____

What is their religious background? (Affiliation, prayer time, symbols, traditions, church/synagogue name, etc. Did they lead any services or sing in the choir?)

_____

_____

_____

What type of music do they enjoy listening to, playing or singing? Do they have any musical talents?

_____

_____

_____

What is their favorite TV program? Movie?

_____

_____

_____

Did they enjoy reading? Which authors, topics, or genres do they prefer? Would they listen to audiobooks or books on tape?

_____

_____

_____

_____

Can they tell the difference between someone on TV and a real person?

_____

_____

Marital status - If married more than once, provide specifics. Include names of spouses, dates of marriage, and other relevant information.

_____

_____

_____

_____

_____

List distinct characteristics about their spouse(s), such as occupations, personality traits or daily routine.

_____

_____

_____

_____

_____

Do they have children? Be sure to include children both living and deceased. Include names, birth dates, and any other relevant information.

_____

_____

_____

_____

_____

Who do they ask for the most? What is their relationship with this person(s)? Describe how that person typically spends their day.

_____

_____

_____

_____

_____

What causes your loved one stress?

_____

_____

_____

_____

What calms them down when they are stressed or agitated?

_____

_____

_____

_____

How long has it been since Parkinson's symptoms first appeared?

_____

Describe how the symptoms of Parkinson's are affecting your loved one.

_____

_____

_____

_____

_____

_____

Have they accepted the Parkinson's?

_____

_____

What activities do they feel they can no longer participate in as a result of the Parkinson's disease?

_____

_____

_____

_____

What specific activities did they enjoy prior to Parkinson's diagnosis?

_____

_____

_____

_____

Are they participating less frequently with family and friends? Can you identify why?

_____

_____

_____

_____

_____

Other information that would help to bring joy to your loved one.

_____

_____

_____

_____

_____

_____

_____

_____

_____

_____

_____

_____

_____

_____

_____

_____

_____

_____

_____

**Note: This form includes questions that are being asked in case your loved one has the dementia symptoms that are caused by their Parkinson's disease.

Functional Levels

In addition to the information gathered in the Personal History Form, which tells everyone what your loved one enjoys, who they are, and what their personal preferences might be, we also need to look at your loved one's functional level. This will allow you to plan activities that your loved one can accomplish. Furthermore, in addition to the Hoehn and Yahr Scale for Parkinson's that we mentioned in Chapter 1, we must also look at functional levels in case your loved one has developed dementia due to Parkinson's.

Level 1

Your loved one has good social skills. They are able to communicate. They are alert and oriented to person, place, and time, and they have a long attention span.

Level 2

Your loved one has less social skills, and their verbal skills may be impaired as well. Your loved one may have some behavior symptoms. They may need something to do, and may have an increased energy level, but they have a shorter attention span.

Level 3

Your loved one has less social skills. Their verbal skills are even more impaired than they were at Level 2. They are also easily distracted. Your loved one may have some visual/spatial perception and balance concerns, and they need maximum assistance with their care.

Level 4

Your loved one has a low energy level, nonverbal communication skills, and they rarely initiate contact with others, however, they may respond if given time and cues.

Chapter 4

Second Pillar of Activities: Communicating and Motivating for Success

Communicating is vital to your success in engaging in an activity with your loved one. Good communication is the Second Pillar of Activities. The key to effective communication is listening attentively and using communication techniques that provide an open, nonthreatening environment for your loved one. Verbal as well as nonverbal communication will play a role in your ability to successfully engage your loved one. How you listen and try to communicate can either enhance and encourage communication or shut down communication altogether. You need to assess your listening and communication style objectively and be able to assess the styles of other caregivers and family members working with your loved one.

Verbal Communication

Communication is simply an interactive process where information is exchanged. More importantly, though, communication is a way to connect with another person. How well you connect depends on your ability to respond appropriately and give feedback on something that was communicated, as well as having good listening skills.

Verbal Approaches for Good Communication

- Use exact, short, positive phrases. Repeat twice if necessary.

- Speak slowly.

- Allow time for the person to answer.

- Give one instruction at a time.

- Use a warm, gentle tone of voice.

- There is no need to shout, unless the individual also has a hearing impairment.

- Since the person may not be able to see you because of a visual impairment, be sure to use verbal cues to let them know you are engaged.

- Talk to them like an adult.

- Only use words your loved one is familiar with.

Verbal Communication Tips

- Make your presence known when entering a room by either saying hello or identifying yourself.

- Identify yourself. Do not assume the person knows or remembers who you are.

- If there are others present, address the person by name so there is no confusion as to whom you are speaking.

- Be sure to indicate the end of a conversation, and ensure your loved one knows when you leave so that they aren't left talking to an empty space.

- Speak directly to your loved one.

- Always answer questions, and be specific or descriptive in your responses.

- When giving directions, make them as clear as possible.

- When speaking with other caregivers or family members about your loved one while they are present, make sure the conversation is respectful of your loved one. They may move or speak slowly, but assume that they hear everything.

Nonverbal Communication

Although it may seem that most communication happens verbally, research has shown that actually most communication occurs nonverbally. Facial expressions, eye contact, gestures, art, and music, and even the amount of physical space between you and your loved one are nonverbal ways to communicate. Nonverbal communication can go a long way to convey your message and make your connection stronger, but it can also undercut your attempts to communicate if your nonverbal cues contradict your intention or send mixed signals.

Even if your loved one is experiencing vision loss due to Parkinson's, your efforts to communicate positively through nonverbal cues and signals do matter.

Remember, too, that the effects of Parkinson's can make it difficult for your loved one to communicate their feelings or reaction to something you are trying to tell them.

The key elements to consider regarding how you communicate nonverbally include:

Facial Expressions

Be aware of what your facial expressions are conveying to your loved one. Your mood will be mirrored.

Eye Contact

Ensure that you have made eye contact with your loved one and that their attention is focused on you and what you are saying.

Gestures and Touch

Calmly use nonverbal signs such as pointing, waving, and other hand gestures in combination with what you are saying.

Tone of Voice

The inflection in your voice helps your loved one relate to the words you are saying.

Body Language

Be aware of the position of your hands and arms when talking to your loved one.

Note: When communicating with your loved one, be mindful that their body language may not fully tell how they feel or what they are trying to express because of rigidity or slow movement. Your loved one, however, will read your body language.

Nonverbal Communication Tips

- Always approach your loved one from the front before speaking to them.

- Smile and extend your hand as to shake their hand. Use touch where welcomed.

- Be at eye level with the person you are talking to.

- Use nonverbal gestures along with words.

- Give nonverbal praises such as smiles and head nods.

- Be an active listener.

- Make sure that all caregivers give your loved one the opportunity and time to speak.

Approaches to Successful Communication and Activities

Be Calm

Always approach your loved one in a relaxed and calm demeanor. Remember, your mood will be mirrored by your loved one. Smiles are contagious.

Be Flexible

There is no right or wrong way of completing a task. Offer praise and encouragement for the effort your loved one puts into a task. If you see your loved one becoming overwhelmed or frustrated, stop the task, and re-approach at another time.

Be Nonresistive

Don't force tasks on your loved one. Adults do not want to be told, "No!" or told what to do. The power of suggestion goes a long way, and you get more with an ounce of sugar than you do a pound of vinegar.

Be Guiding, but Not Controlling

Always use a soft, gentle approach, and remember your tone of voice. Your facial expressions must match the words you are saying.

Barriers to Good Communication

There are generally two barriers that negatively affect communication with your loved one. Here are some tips on how to eliminate negative barriers.

Caregiver Barriers

- Slow down when speaking. Use a calm tone of voice, and be aware of your hand movements.

- Never be demanding or commanding.

- Never argue with a person with impaired cognition. You will never win the argument.

- Enter their world. Live their truth.

- Do not offer long explanations when answering questions.

Environmental Barriers

- Minimize noise from air conditioners and home appliances.

- Turn off the TV if it is on in the same room where you are trying to talk.

- Be aware of outside traffic noise.

- Check your loved one's hearing aid battery, and make sure that it is not whistling.

- Adjust the lighting in the room. If the lighting in a room makes seeing even more difficult for someone with limited vision, they may be more focused on trying to see rather than on communicating with you.

Validation of "Living their Truth" as a Tool to Communicating with Someone who has Dementia

For those we care for who have dementia, R.O.S. teaches validation as part of the communication process.

Validation encourages caregivers to enter their loved one's world and experience what they are experiencing—by living in that moment with them. In other words, rather than correcting your loved one in an effort to get them to understand that what they believe is real is only real in their mind, you respond to them where they are. For example, say that you find your loved one crying because their mother died a couple of days ago. You know that your loved one's mother passed away 50 years ago, not a couple of days ago. It does no good to get into an argument about when the mother died. The kindest approach to take is for you to acknowledge and validate your loved one's sorrow and loss as they are experiencing it and believing it. Your role when working with your loved one is best expressed by author Jolene Brackey, who preaches that caregivers should take every opportunity to create moments of joy.

Many people struggle with the use of validation. There is a concern that it might appear as if you are lying to your loved one or doing them harm by not keeping them oriented to the truth. In fact, you are not lying to your loved one. You are simply meeting your loved one where they are at this moment and accepting that this is part of the illness.

Communication and Behavior

Behaviors are a means to communicate when words are no longer effective. When someone has difficulty or is unable to speak, the easiest way to communicate and express feelings, whether they are positive or negative, is through behavior. It might help to think of a bright young toddler who has a limited vocabulary, and so he expresses his wants and needs through what might be either good or bad behavior. With Parkinson's, it can become just as difficult for an adult to communicate their wants and needs. Caregivers must uncover the meaning behind the behaviors, and put a plan into effect to manage those needs. Be a detective.

Aggressive Behaviors

Aggressive behaviors can include hitting, angry outbursts, obscenities, yelling, racial insults, making inappropriate sexual comments, and/or biting. Trying to communicate with or provide care to a person who is aggressive can be stressful and even frightening for caregivers.

The following are some of the personal and environmental factors that may lead your loved one to show aggressive behavior.

- Too much noise or overstimulation
- Cluttered environment
- Uncomfortable room temperatures
- Basic needs not being met: hunger, thirst, needing to use the bathroom, needing comfort
- Pain
- Fear, anxiety or confusion
- Communication barriers

- Fear or anxiety from not recognizing their surroundings

- Caregiver's mood

- Feeling that they are being rushed

- Difficulty seeing activity or materials of activity, which prevents them from participating

- Lack of independence

Interventions to Mitigate Aggressive Behaviors

- Communicate for success.

- Reminisce with your loved one about specific details of their past.

- Validate and support their feelings.

- Remain calm, and speak in a soft tone.

- Find items that they find comfort in, e.g., a picture of the family.

- Provide consistent caregivers and schedules. Stick to your loved one's routine.

- Engage in recreational activities that match their abilities and interests, as tolerated.

- Break down instructions into one-step increments.

- Identify the triggers of the aggression. Be a detective. There is never a behavior that just occurs.

- Keep an ongoing dialogue between family members and caregivers over any noted changes in patterns or behaviors.

- Help your loved one to slow down and relax.

- Play or listen to music your loved one enjoys for its calming effects.

- Use spiritual support if this is important to your loved one.

Chapter 5

Third Pillar of Activities:
Customary Routines and Preferences

Maintaining your loved one's customary routines and basing activities on your loved one's preferences is the Third Pillar of Activities. Engaging your loved one in activities that promote a sense of accomplishment, provide opportunities for communicating and sharing, and help to maintain and improve functional and cognitive abilities can and should be part of each day's routine. The question should not be, "When should I do activities?" The focus should be on making each and every interaction memorable and always focusing on your loved one as an individual.

In helping you to develop a daily plan of care for your loved one, we will be discussing two areas: Daily Customary Routine and Activity Preferences. The goal is to gain from your loved one's perspective how important certain aspects of care/activity are to them as an individual.

Daily Customary Routine

Your loved one has distinct lifestyle preferences and routines that should be preserved to the greatest extent possible. All reasonable accommodation should be made to maintain your loved one's lifestyle preferences. Perhaps for years prior to the onset of symptoms, your loved one woke up every Sunday morning, made a cup of coffee, and sat down to read the newspaper. They took their coffee with two teaspoons of sugar and sat at the head of the kitchen table to read the newspaper. You should try to find ways to keep those activities a part of your loved one's routine. If the disease has progressed to the point that they cannot enjoy their Sunday morning coffee routine on their own, what could you or other caregivers do to help them maintain at least some of that routine?

Your loved one's ability to do many things independently, abilities that were taken for granted before Parkinson's, might become diminished or lost due to the effects of Parkinson's. With your help, however, allowing your loved one to preserve as much of their routine as possible will go a long way to improving and maintaining their confidence, mood, and overall well-being.

Not accommodating your loved one's lifestyle preferences and routine can contribute to a depressed mood and increased behavior issues. When a person feels like their control has been removed and that their preferences are being disregarded and not respected, it can be demoralizing.

Activity Preferences

Activities are a way for individuals to establish meaning in their lives. The need for enjoyable activities does not lessen or change based on their age or health needs. The only thing that changes is the level of assistance they might need to engage in those pursuits.

A lack of opportunity to engage in meaningful and enjoyable activities can result in boredom, depression, and behavioral disturbances.

Individuals vary in the activities they prefer, reflecting unique personalities, past interests, perceived environmental constraints, religious and cultural background, and changing physical and mental abilities. We as family caregivers have a great opportunity to empower a loved one to still see that they possess many great talents and abilities. By modifying or adapting an activity to allow them to engage at an independent level, you are restoring their self-esteem and self-worth.

Chapter 6

Fourth Pillar of Activities:
Planning and Executing Activities

Planning and executing activities is the Fourth Pillar of Activities. Activities occur all day, every day. While certainly some activities can be spontaneous, most people find that the best activities are planned ahead. Spending some time to plan activities helps to ensure that they are appropriate for your loved one and offer the greatest opportunity for success. Please note again that schedules, routines, and plans should be followed. However, they may need to be adapted due to the progression of the disease or specific symptoms your loved one may be experiencing on a particular day.

As you plan your loved one's activities as part of their customary routine, you need to consider how an activity fits within the following criteria:

- Person Appropriate—Desires and Preferences
- Person Appropriate—Abilities and Functional Levels

Person Appropriate— Desires and Preferences

Person appropriate refers to the idea that each person has a personal identity and history. Everyone has unique desires and preferences, and a "person appropriate" activity is one that is designed with an individual's preferences in mind. It also means that the primary caregiver has to make sure that all caregivers understand the elements and purpose of each specific activity. Lesson Plans are invaluable tools to communicate clearly and consistently to all caregivers the elements of an activity.

Remember our gardening example? Four people said that they enjoy "gardening," but to each of them "gardening" meant something different. The example helps to illustrate how important it is when planning activities that you ensure that the activity is person appropriate and is based on the specific desires and preferences of your loved one.

Person Appropriate— Abilities and Functional Levels

This concept is also based on the idea that each person has a personal identity and history, but it also takes into account the varying functional levels at which a person may be able to participate in an activity. The effects of age, declining health, Parkinson's and other diseases on a person's physical and mental abilities, at some point may mean that while many activities can still be performed, some activities may be facilitated through certain modifications, e.g., by using adaptive equipment. Based on your loved one's functional level and abilities, some activities may also be done as a group activity. This creates an opportunity for socialization, interaction, and conversation between you and your loved one. Remember our gardening example when looking at personal preference. Let's use that example again to look at person appropriate based on abilities.

- Person 1—Enjoys going outside, cutting the grass, trimming the hedges, and weed whacking. Anything less would not meet his preference.

  As the disease has progressed, Person 1 is no longer able to perform the cutting and the trimming, but may be able to supervise or offer advice to someone doing those things. In this case, the outdoor activity can be discussed, planned, and executed together.

- Person 2—Enjoys getting in the flower beds, planting flowers and vegetables, and tending to her garden on her hands and knees each day for an hour.

As this person's disease has progressed, Person 2 finds that she is no longer able to get down in the garden to plant. Adaptive equipment such as the Gardening Board insert from the R.O.S. Legacy System can be used to allow her to continue to plant seeds. The planted seeds can be placed in her room so that she can water them and watch them grow. Once the seeds sprout, they can then be planted outside with assistance from others.

- Person 3—Enjoys indoor plants, propagating plants, and watering and caring for plants daily.

Person 3 can no longer move easily through the house to water each plant. In this case, a watering station can be set up in a central location, such as on the kitchen table. A caregiver can bring each plant to the table so that each plant is watered, providing Person 3 the opportunity to still participate in something he enjoys.

- Person 4—Enjoys arranging flowers in vases for tables.

Parkinson's has left Person 4 without the ability to grasp or arrange flowers herself. She is still able to participate, however, by being given the opportunity to choose the vase and the flowers and directing where and how the flowers should be arranged.

The Lesson Plan

A Lesson Plan is a tool that you can use to help plan activities. A good Lesson Plan consists of a list of items needed to complete the activity, clear instructions, and room to record any and all observations regarding your loved one's participation and engagement. All caregivers should use the Lesson Plan to stay up-to-date and informed as to your loved one's ability to participate in an activity. Over time, your loved one's interest or ability to engage in a particular activity may change, so we suggest using the activity Lesson Plan to document everything you or any other caregiver observes each time you engage with your loved one.

As your loved one's abilities and responses change, those changes will dictate how you modify an activity to meet their current needs and abilities. The Lesson Plan is an ever-changing document. It is meant to be written on to note the changes you made to the original plan so that the family member or caregiver working with your loved one next can follow your modifications in the hopes of recreating a positive experience.

Items in the Lesson Plan

Date

Document the date the program is used with your loved one.

Program Name

You can rename the program if you or your loved one prefer.

Objective of Activity

Our goal is to provide meaningful activities. People have a need to be productive, and they want to engage in something with a purpose. List the objectives of the program.

Materials

List of suggested materials to use with this program.

Prerequisite Skills

Skills your loved one needs to participate in this program.

Activity Outline

Step-by-step instructions to complete this program.

When you or a family member are conducting an activity with your loved one, documenting results and responses is critical to identifying ways to improve activity programs for your loved one. Items to document should include:

- Verbal cues, physical assistance or modifications you required for this activity.

- How your loved one responded to this program.

- Whether your loved one enjoyed this activity. What did they like or dislike about the activity?

- Whether the activity was successful at distracting or eliminating a negative behavior. Why and how was it successful?

A blank template is included on the next page to give you an example of what a Lesson Plan looks like.

Note: Make sure caregivers and family members are consistent with the type of verbal cues, physical assistance or modifications that produce positive results.

Lesson Plan Blank Example

Date	Program Name

Objective of Activity

Materials

Prerequisite Skills

Room Lighting

Activity Outline

Evaluation

Chapter 7

Leisure Activity Categories, Types, Tips, and Suggestions

Activity Categories

There are as many different possibilities for activities as there are individuals to create them for. To keep things simple, we place activities into three general categories: Maintenance Activities, Supportive Activities, and Empowering Activities.

Maintenance Activities

Maintenance activities are traditional activities that help a person to maintain physical, cognitive, social, spiritual, and emotional health.

Examples include: using manipulative games such as those in the R.O.S. Legacy System, craft and art activities, attending church services, working trivia and crossword puzzles like the *How Much Do You Know About* puzzles, taking a walk, and tai chi.

Supportive Activities

If your loved one has a lower tolerance for traditional activities, supportive activities provide a comfortable environment while providing stimulation or solace.

Examples include: listening to and singing music, hand massages, relaxation activities such as aromatherapy, meditation, and bird-watching.

Empowering Activities

Empowering activities help your loved one build and maintain self-respect by offering opportunities for self-expression and exercising responsibility.

Examples include: cooking, making memory boxes, and folding laundry.

General Activity Tips

It is likely that your loved one will need some level of assistance from you when engaging in activities. Because one of the key goals of doing activities is to foster a sense of accomplishment and independence, we offer the following tips to help you anticipate some of the things that might come up in the course of engaging your loved one, to increase your loved one's chances for success, and to help make the experience a positive one for both of you.

Travel Tips for Moving from Room to Room or Place to Place

- When escorting your loved one, ask them if they need assistance. If they do not request any assistance, walk side by side or a half step behind in case they experience freezing or fall.

- If your loved one experiences freezing, please remember your communication techniques—be calm, be flexible, be guiding, but not controlling. There is no need to yell or startle them while they are working through taking a step. If you are in public, yelling may draw unwanted attention to them, causing them to focus on avoiding embarrassment rather than on taking a step.

- If your loved one does require some assistance, offer your arm to be held onto or interlocked with. Find the easiest and most comfortable way to walk together. Walk side by side or a half pace ahead while providing verbal cues about the environment.

- Announce when you are approaching doorways, stairs, and ramps.

- Avoid puddles, snowbanks, and other natural barriers.

- Avoid cracked tile, untacked throw rugs, and protruding floorboards.

Writing and Coloring Activity Tips

- If your loved one has trouble holding a pen or pencil, wrap foam around the shaft of the pen to help your loved one's grip. You can try cutting a small piece from a foam noodle used for swimming to fit on the writing tool.

- Reduce glare and shadowing by positioning a chair and table so any natural light is behind them instead of coming at them from the front.

- To prevent shadows, place lamps on the opposite side of the hand being used. Locate the bottom edge of the lampshade just below eye level.

- Shiny paper can increase glare, so it is best to use matte paper when reading or writing.

- Use large-print crossword, word search, or word scramble puzzles. See the R.O.S. *How Much Do You Know About* series of e-

Books. If you cannot find these books or other large-print sources, most copiers have the ability to increase the size of the print.

- A dry-erase board or tablet may also be used to practice writing.

** **Note:** Know the type of seating where your loved one is the most comfortable when they are writing, and, if possible, move them to that seat.

** **Note:** If your loved one is seated in a wheelchair, recliner or bed, provide a flat surface that fits in their lap to place paper on.

** **Note:** Your loved one may experience shrinking handwriting due to bradykinesia.

Reading Activity Tips

- Large-print books are available at most bookstores and libraries.

- Read to your loved one or take turns reading to each other.

- Listen to audio tapes and books on CD borrowed from your local library, or from the free Talking Books program sponsored by the National Library Service.

- If your loved one prefers reading to listening, many new mobile devices such as iPads, Kindles, and Nooks all have options to increase the font size and adjust the color contrast.

- Try the Book Strap from the R.O.S. Legacy System to help keep a book and the page in place.

Craft Activity Tips

- Make sure that supplies are easily accessible.

- Empower your loved one by choosing an area of the home where they can most comfortably participate.

  ○ If at a table and in a wheelchair, make sure the wheelchair can fit under the table.

  ○ If in a recliner, use an activity surface that fits comfortably in their lap, and choose an activity that does not have too many pieces that may be hard to keep track of.

- Craft Boxes and Materials

  ○ Place craft activity supplies in boxes clearly labeled with a broad-tipped black marker.

  ○ Group like items for activities together.

  ○ Store materials in different shaped/sized containers.

○ Choose identifying and organizational systems that work best for your loved one.

Game Playing Activity Tips

Playing Cards:

- If needed, use adaptive equipment to place the playing cards in while your loved one is seated at a table.

- The Card Holder Board Insert from the R.O.S. Legacy System allows your loved one to have the card holder in their lap while seated in a recliner or wheelchair.

Puzzles:

- Choose puzzles with larger pieces. These are easier for your loved one to manipulate.

- If your loved one becomes frustrated because puzzle pieces are sliding when being placed, try a magnetic puzzle and a metallic flat surface so the pieces stay in place.

Active Activity Suggestions

Active activities, such as walking, dancing, and stretching, are those that involve using large muscle groups. In addition to the tips we offer for general activities, following are some suggestions for active activities. As you build these activities into your loved one's schedule, please be sure to leave opportunities for rest after or between activities. Depending on the activity or exercise, you, a family member, or a trained professional should always be there to supervise and assist your loved one as needed.

Generally speaking, there are four types of Active Activities: aerobic, strengthening, flexibility, and balance. Any of them can help to improve the quality of life for your loved one.

Aerobic Activities

During aerobic activities, the body's large muscles move in a rhythmic manner for a sustained period of time. Aerobic activities help to maintain or improve cardiovascular health. Objectives of aerobic activities include: improving physical fitness and having positive effects on slowness, stiffness, and mood.

Examples of aerobic activities for your loved one:

- Walking
  - with you, a family member, a friend, or your dog
  - on a treadmill
  - on a gentle hike, in a city park
  - around the shopping mall

- Swimming or water aerobics
  - at your gym or YMCA

- Riding a bike
  - around the neighborhood or on a stationary bike

- Dancing
  - at home with you, a family member, or a friend
  - at a local dance hall, club, or ballet center

- Chair aerobics
  - in your living room following along with a video
  - at your local gym or YMCA

Strengthening Activities

Strengthening activities improve muscle strength, walking speed, posture, and overall physical fitness. The objective of improving muscle strength is to facilitate everyday activities such as getting up from a chair, moving from room to room in the home, and making any task easier to manage.

Examples of strengthening activities for your loved one:

- Weights/resistance
  - free weight activities/exercises
  - elastic bands activities/exercises
  - body weight activities/exercises

- Yard work or gardening

Flexibility Activities

Flexibility or stretching exercises improve mobility, increase range of motion, reduce stiffness, and can help to reduce the risk of injury. Stretching and flexibility activities can improve range of motion, which can affect posture and walking ability, reducing the risk of injury, and making everyday activities easier.

Examples of flexibility activities for your loved one:

- Tai chi
- Gentle stretching
  - In your living room following along with a video
- Yoga, including chair yoga

Balance Activities

Balance activities can improve posture and stability. Preserving your loved one's ability to maintain their balance can help to reduce the likelihood of falling, potentially calm your loved one's fears of falling, and help them generally in performing daily tasks.

Examples of balance activities for your loved one:

- Yoga, including chair yoga
- Tai chi
- At-home balance exercises using
  - A Wii
  - A balance ball or balance pillow

Chapter 8

Activities of Daily Living Tips and Suggestions

Unlike the leisure activities discussed, the activities of daily living covered in this book are necessary activities that are a part of everyday life. The following pages contain tips and suggestions for you to use with your loved one.

Energy Conservation and Rest

Energy conservation and rest are vital for someone with Parkinson's. As the day is scheduled, make sure there are planned periods of rest between activities. Simplifying daily tasks so your loved one uses less energy can help them have more energy to do more activities throughout the day. Look at each activity and decide if the way your loved one has always done the activity is the most efficient and uses the least amount of their energy.

All activities of the day should be planned out—this includes ADLs, leisure activities, chores, and exercise. They should be spaced throughout the day, with the items that require the most energy being accomplished at the time of day your loved one feels the best.

Do not schedule too many things to do in one day, and be prepared to cancel some plans if your loved one is not feeling well or up to it.

If your loved one becomes tired during an activity, let them stop and rest. If your loved one turns a rest period into a nap, be careful not to let them nap too much during the day as they might not be able to sleep at night.

Bathing

Bathing can be a relaxing, enjoyable experience or a time of confrontation and anger. Use a calm approach. Your loved one's "usual" routine is very important.

Safety and Preparation

- Water temperature should range from 110-115 degrees Fahrenheit maximum to prevent burning or skin injury.

- Hot water can cause fatigue.

- The floor of tub needs to be slip proof. Use a rubber mat that doesn't slide, or use permanent nonslip decals.

- Place a nonskid rug on the floor outside the tub to prevent slipping.

- Install grab bars.

- Do not use bath oils.

Bathing—Know Your Loved One

- Are they accustomed to a bath or shower?

- Can they get into a bath or shower without assistance?

- Can they soap their body or wash their hair themselves?

- Can they dry themselves with a towel, with simple tricks such as sewing straps onto the towel to make the towel easier to hold?

- If they need help, who is your loved one the most comfortable with when needing assistance bathing?

Bathing—Communicating and Motivating

- Don't ask if they want to bathe. Simply say in an easy, friendly voice, "Bath time."

- Use short, simple sentences.

- Look directly at your loved one.

- Always smile, and talk calmly and gently.

- Do not argue, or try to explain "why."

Bathing—Customary Routines and Preferences

- What time of day does your loved one normally bathe?

- How often did your loved one bathe?

- What is the process that works for you and your loved one when it is time to bathe? Make sure all caregivers know each detail of the process.

  For example, is the water turned on and running prior to your loved one entering the tub? Is a towel placed on a shower chair that your loved one may use so that chill on their bottom is removed when they sit?

  Whatever the process, take it one step at a time, following their normal bathing routine. For example, wash their hair first and then body, or soak for 10 minutes before washing.

- When assisting your loved one, have a towel ready to put over their shoulders or on their lap so they feel less exposed.

Bathing—Planning and Executing

- Have all care items and tools ready prior to starting the bath process.

  ◦ A shower chair if necessary

  ◦ A handheld hose for showering and bathing

  ◦ A long-handled sponge or scrubbing brush if they would like to scrub themselves

  ◦ Sponges with soap inside or a soft soap applicator instead of bar soap. Bar soap can easily slip out of your loved one's hand.

- Have a towel and clothing prepared for when the bath is finished.

- A second towel can be placed on the back of a chair to allow your loved one to dry their back by rubbing on the towel.

- Use a terry cloth robe instead of a towel to dry off.

Other Bathroom & Grooming Activities

Brushing Teeth

- If your loved one has also developed dementia with their Parkinson's and assistance is needed, start with step-by-step directions. This might not be as simple as you think. Take a moment and think of all of the steps necessary to brush your teeth, from walking into the bathroom, to finding the toothpaste in the drawer and removing the cap, to rinsing their mouth once they have finished brushing. Depending on your loved one's level of dementia, it might be easier to show them.

- For family members at home, brush your teeth at the same time.

- Use positive reinforcement, and compliment your loved one on the good job they are doing.

- Help your loved one to clean their dentures as needed.

Shaving

- Encourage a male to shave.

- Use an electric razor for safety.

- If they need assistance, please provide it.

- Give positive feedback, and do not verbally correct.

Makeup

- If your loved one had been accustomed to wearing makeup, there is no reason for this to stop. If she shows interest or a desire to wear makeup, encourage her to do so, and offer assistance to apply it if needed.

Hair

- Try to maintain hairstyle and care as your loved one did.

- Explain each step simply before you do anything to reduce any anxiety.

Nails

- Keep nails clean and trimmed. Be gentle while trimming your loved one's nails. Be mindful of how and where you place their fingers and arms.

- Offer to polish your loved one's nails.

- When polishing, engage your loved one in conversation.

- If your loved one had a normal/weekly schedule for nail care prior to the onset of Parkinson's, please try to maintain that schedule.

Toileting or Using the Bathroom

- Learn your loved one's individual habits and routines for using the toilet. This might not be something that you know and is part of the changing roles.

- Toilet routinely on rising, before and after meals, and at bedtime, at minimum.

- If your loved one is having trouble communicating, please watch for agitation, pulling at their clothes, or restless walking or pacing. This may be an indication that they need to go to the bathroom.

- Assist with clothing as needed, and be positive and pleasant while assisting.

- Provide verbal cues and instructions as needed. Be guiding, but not controlling.

Clothing

Clothing—Know Your Loved One

- Daily clothing choices should remain as they had been and based on their available wardrobe during the initial stages of the disease.

- As their Parkinson's disease progresses, changes will have to be made. Clothes need to be comfortable and easy to remove, especially to go to bathroom.

- Choose clothes that are loose fitting and have elastic waistbands.

- For convenience, choose wraparound clothing instead of the pullover type.

- If possible, choose clothing that opens in the front, not the back. This prevents your loved one from having to reach behind themselves and allows them to maintain the feeling of independence from dressing themselves.

- When purchasing new clothes, look for clothing with large, flat buttons, Velcro closures or zippers.

- To assist your loved one with zipping pants or a jacket, attach a zipper pull or leather loop on the end of the zipper.

- Choose slip-on shoes.

Clothing—Communicating and Motivating

- Use short, simple sentences.

- Provide verbal cues/instructions as needed.

- Always smile.

- Talk calmly and gently.

- Do not argue, or try to explain "why."

Clothing—Routines and Preferences

- Have a friendly discussion each evening about the next day's schedule and what your loved one may want to wear.

- If your loved one also has dementia, changes will have to be made as the dementia progresses. You may have to limit the choice of clothing, and leave only two outfits in their room at a time.

- If your loved one wants to wear the same thing every day, and if you can afford it, buy three or four sets of the same clothing.

Clothing—Planning and Executing

- Clothes should be laid out according to what goes on first.

- Do not use panty hose, knee-high nylons, tight socks, or high heels.

- Make sure that items are not inside out and that buttons, zips, and fasteners are all undone before handing the clothes to your loved one.

Dressing

Dressing—Know Your Loved One

Initially, your loved one may just need verbal cues and instructions on dressing. Please remember to allow them to dress themselves as long as possible so they can maintain a sense of dignity and independence. As the primary caregiver, you will have to be the judge as to when all caregivers need to begin assisting your loved one with dressing.

Dressing—Communicating and Motivating

- Use short, simple sentences, and provide instruction as needed.

- If your loved one is confused, give instructions in very short steps, such as, "Now put your arm through the sleeve." It may help to use actions to demonstrate these instructions.

- Offer praise. Dressing really can be a pretty challenging task even under the best circumstances.

- Always smile.

- Speak calmly and gently.

- Do not argue, or try to explain "why."

- Remember to ask your loved one if they would like to go to the toilet before getting dressed.

Dressing—Routines and Preferences

- Does your loved one get dressed first thing in the morning—before breakfast or after breakfast?

- Does your loved one change into pajamas right before bed or after dinner?

- Try to maintain your loved one's preferred routine for as long as possible.

- Little things matter. For example, they may like to put on all of their underwear before putting on anything else.

Dressing—Planning and Executing

- Think about privacy—make sure that blinds or curtains are closed and that no one will walk in and disturb your loved one while they are dressing.

- Make sure the room is warm.

- Hand your loved one a single item at a time.

- Let your loved one get dressed while sitting in a chair that has armrests. This will help them keep their balance.

- If it is helpful, have your loved one use a dressing stick to get a coat or shirt on or off.

- If your loved one wants to put their pants on without help from you, suggest they roll from side to side to get the pants over their hips. They can try doing this while sitting in a chair or lying down on a bed.

- If needed, have your loved one use a button hook to button clothing.

If mistakes are made—for example, by putting something on the wrong way—be tactful, or find a way for both of you to laugh about it.

** **Note:** Wearing several layers of thin clothing rather than one thick layer can be helpful. With layers, your loved one will be able to remove a layer if it gets too warm.

Remember that your loved one will get to a point where they no longer will be able to tell you if they are too hot or cold, so keep an eye out for signs of discomfort.

Eating

Eating—Know Your Loved One

- Keep long-standing personal preferences in mind when preparing food. However, be aware that your loved one may suddenly develop new food preferences or reject foods that they enjoyed in the past.

- Can your loved one feed themselves?

- Does your loved one have a visual impairment that may affect their ability to see their meal or drink? Due to normal changes in our eyesight as we age, eating and dining may offer additional challenges.

Eating—Communicating and Motivating

- Use short, simple sentences.

- Provide verbal cues and instructions as needed.

- Give your loved one your full attention.

- Always smile, and talk calmly and gently.

- Be guiding, but not controlling.

Eating—Routines and Preferences

- No matter the time of day they eat breakfast, lunch and dinner, be consistent every day.

- Offer snacks throughout the day.

- Limit distractions. Serve meals in quiet surroundings, away from the television and other activities.

- Factor into the overall schedule of the day that it may take an hour or longer to finish each meal or snack.

Note: Your loved one's sense of taste may change. They might not enjoy food that they have eaten for years. Make note of any changes in your loved one's food preferences on the Personal History Form.

Eating—Planning and Executing

This simple, everyday activity requires maneuvering objects, a skill that many of us may take for granted. You and your loved one will need to develop techniques that work for your loved one.

- It is completely appropriate to ask your loved one if they would like any assistance.

- Offer to dish the food onto your loved one's plate, if needed.

- When cutting food, make sure the pieces are small enough for your loved one to chew and swallow easily.

- Use appropriate lighting for each meal.

  ○ Reduce glare by having your loved one sit with the sunlight behind them when eating.

  ○ Use overhead lighting that illuminates the entire dining space and makes objects visible, as well as reduces shadows or reflections.

- Create clear visual distinctions between the table, dishes, and food.

  - Use solid colors with no distracting patterns.

  - When pouring a light-colored drink, such as milk, use a dark glass.

  - When pouring a dark-colored drink, such as cola, use a white glass.

  - Avoid clear glasses. They can disappear from view.

  - Use white dishes when eating dark-colored food, and use dark dishes when eating light-colored food.

  - To make dishes easier to find on the table, use a tablecloth or placemats that are the opposite color of the dishes.

** **Note:** Fiesta ware colors (yellow/tangerine) contrast with most foods so they can be easily seen and will enhance visual perception.

Setting the Table

If your loved one is in the early stages of Parkinson's and can feed themselves while sitting at a table, keep these tips in mind.

- Have your loved one help in the kitchen and set the table if they are able.

- Set the table as your loved one is used to every day.

- Use a nonskid mat for objects placed on the table.

- Use a plate with a raised lip to prevent food from spilling.

- Use adaptive utensils if needed.

- Use a long straw with a non-spill cup, or use a plastic mug with a large handle.

- Set each place setting in the same way for every meal.

- Place the knife and spoon to the right of the plate.

- Place the fork and napkin to the left of the plate.

- Place the glass or cup above the plate to the right or left, depending on whether your loved one is left- or right-handed.

- Decide how to set the rest of the table— main dish, side dishes, seasonings, and condiments. Do it the same way each day.

Other Meal Considerations

- Your loved one might not be able to tell if something is too hot to eat or drink. Always test the temperature of foods and beverages before serving.

- Make meals an enjoyable social event so everyone looks forward to the experience.

- Clean up spills immediately.

- Let your loved one know it is okay to rest their elbows on the table to provide more motion at the wrist and hand.

Meals and Dementia

Eating a meal can be a challenge for your loved one with Parkinson's. If your loved one also has dementia, you may want to consider a few additional options that can help to reduce mealtime issues and problems.

Meal Preparation for Someone with Mild Dementia

If your loved one wants to assist in making a meal:

- Make sure your cabinets are organized with each item labeled with large, easy-to-see labels.

- Use simple step-by-step written or verbal instructions.

- For safety's sake, you or another caregiver must perform tasks like cutting, which require the use of a sharp knife, or cooking on a stove, or baking in an oven.

- When using a stove top, use the back burners, and turn the handles inward toward the back of the stove to avoid any potential grabbing of the pots or pans.

- If you are not there to supervise because you have to go to work:

  ○ Avoid planning meals that require use of the stove. Your loved one might not remember to turn off the stove and might not be able to distinguish between a pot that is hot or cold.

  ○ Lay out the ingredients of a meal on the counter or in the refrigerator in labeled containers in the order that your loved one will use them (similar to laying out their clothes at night).

○ Transfer bulk items, including milk, from a larger container or jug to a smaller container that will be easier to lift and pour.

Meal Preparation for Someone with Higher Level Dementia

- Try to eat all meals seated at a kitchen or dining room table or a chair with a serving tray.

- Avoid serving meals in bed if possible. Let the bed be only for sleeping.

Activities of daily living can be challenging as your loved one's disease progresses, but they can be accomplished. Making sure that all caregivers know your loved one, their routine, and the game plan for any activity will help you and your loved one to be successful.

Chapter 9

Home Preparation

Whether you live in a house, an apartment, or an independent living facility, you and your loved one need to feel comfortable, capable, and safe. This is a key foundational piece of preparing to have your loved one engage in any activity. The following are general tips that caregivers and family members can use to prepare the home to accommodate your loved one's needs as their Parkinson's disease progresses.

General Organization and Environment

When organizing your loved one's environment, be sure to do it <u>with</u> them. What works for you, might not work for your loved one.

- Assign everything to a place in the home. Always put items back in their place after using them in order to avoid clutter.

- Remove objects frequently left on the floor, such as shoes, bags, and boxes. They should be placed in their designated areas of the home. If left out, they can be a tripping hazard.

- Use extension cords sparingly, and always secure them out of the places where people walk. Bundle all the cords, and secure them to the wall instead of the floor.

- Organize like objects in the same area whenever possible so that they are easily located.

- Remove and avoid clutter on desks, tables, and countertops, and in cabinets and closets. This makes it easier to locate and reach specific items.

- Avoid using throw rugs. Although they can make for good identifying markers or nice decorative pieces, they can also be a tripping hazard when your loved one is moving from room to room. If you must use them, opt for slide-resistant rugs that can be taped or tacked down.

- Install handrails where possible for easier independent movement from one room to the next.

- Leave doors fully opened or closed. Make sure the doors open easily and smoothly, and that doorknobs are securely fastened to the door.

- Identify and address flooring issues. Check every floor, walkway, threshold, and entry. Remove or fix loose floorboards, uneven tiles, loose nails, or carpeting that has bunched up over time.

Furniture

- Make sure there is enough room to move around. If possible, place furniture pieces 5½ feet from each other so your loved one can move comfortably around the room, especially if they are in a wheelchair.

- Where possible, arrange your furniture so outlets are easily accessible for lamps and other electrical items without the need for extension cords.

- Use chairs with straight backs, armrests, and firm seats. Where possible, add firm cushions to existing pieces to add height. This will make it easier for your loved one to sit down and get up.

Lighting

Depending on your loved one's vision, Parkinson's symptoms, or individual preference, you may find it necessary to modify existing lighting in the home. These changes could be key in your loved one's safety and ability to perform tasks independently.

- Fluorescent lighting can contribute to an increase in glare. Try different types of lightbulbs to see which is most comfortable for your loved one.

- Keep all rooms evenly lit and the lighting level consistent throughout the home so shadows and dangerous bright spots are eliminated.

- Make sure light switches, pull cords, and lamps are easily accessible for your loved one in case they are in a wheelchair.

- If possible, purchase touch lamps or those that can be turned on or off by sound.

- Be certain that all stairwells are well lit and have handrails.

- Depending on the individual, additional task lighting may be necessary in certain areas of the home.

- Additional lighting for closets and smaller areas may be helpful. Battery-operated push lights are a good option.

Glare

Glare can be caused by sunlight or light from a lamp. When light hits a shiny surface, such as a magazine page or even a wall painted with high-gloss paint, the resulting glare can make it difficult for someone with low vision to see.

Sunglasses can be beneficial both indoors and outside for someone who is light sensitive. Offer your loved one an opportunity to try different lens colors to see which works best for them.

- Sunlight can fill the room with light without producing glare. Adjust sunlight coming through windows by using mini blinds and altering their position throughout the day. If mini blinds are not available, use sheer curtains to diffuse the light.

- Be aware when placing mirrors in a room. Mirrors placed across from larger windows can significantly increase the amount of light in a room. This could be beneficial for someone who prefers the additional light.

- Cover bare lightbulbs with shades.

- Position chairs and tables so that when your loved one is sitting on a chair or at a table, they are not having to look directly at the light coming from a window.

- Cover or remove shiny/reflective surfaces such as floors and tabletops.

Color Contrasts

Using contrast is a good strategy if your loved one has a visual impairment due to Parkinson's or for another reason. The more contrast, the easier it is to find and use objects or activity items around the house.

- Put light-colored objects against a dark background.

- Avoid upholstery with patterns for seated activities. Stripes, plaids, and checks can be visually confusing.

- Opt for solid-colored tables and countertops in a neutral tone. Countertops with busy patterns can make it difficult to locate items and can be more difficult to keep clean.

- In a room with mostly dark tones, place light-colored pillows or chairs in strategic places to help your loved one find things and get around easily.

- Put contrasting stripes on the edges of stairs to make each stair visible and to prevent the stairs from disappearing from view.

Chapter 10

Review

The motor and nonmotor effects of Parkinson's disease, and their progression, vary with each individual. Freezing, tremors, bradykinesia, loss of balance, diminished vision, and depression are just some of the challenges of living with Parkinson's. Learning to live with and coming to accept the changes can be difficult, not only for the person who has Parkinson's, but for family and friends, as well. As your loved one's primary caregiver, you are in a unique position to understand and see that your loved one's needs are being met. By taking advantage of offers of assistance from family members, friends, and others who are in a position to carry some of the responsibilities of caregiver, the work of caring for your loved one at home can be made a bit easier. One of the keys to making it all work is ensuring that all caregivers are working from the same page. Reading this book is a good first step in reaching that goal.

There are many things to consider and do when caring for a loved one at home. The home must be a safe place for your loved one. We offer many suggestions for preparing your home so that it is a safe environment, but ultimately the decisions on best preparations and changes needed for your loved one are up to you. We offer guidance for communicating with your loved one, when communication is made more difficult by the effects of Parkinson's.

We encourage you to make every effort to identify, plan, and incorporate activities for your loved one into each day. Meaningful, person-appropriate activities can improve the quality of life for both you and your loved one. There are so many benefits to an Activity Program for your loved one, and you have the opportunity to enjoy them all. If you keep in mind our Four Pillars of Activities as you consider the many activity possibilities, you will be able to choose and implement the activities that are best suited for your loved one.

Here, again, are the Four Pillars of Activities.

First Pillar of Activities: Know your Loved One—Information Gathering and Assessment

Have a Personal History Form completed. Know them—who they are, who they were, and what their functional abilities are today. Make sure all caregivers know this as well.

Second Pillar of Activities: Communicating and Motivating for Success

Communication is key. Each caregiver must know how to effectively communicate with your loved one and be consistent with techniques.

Third Pillar of Activities: Customary Routines and Preferences

As best as possible, maintain a routine and daily plan based on your loved one's needs and preferences.

Fourth Pillar of Activities: Planning and Executing Activities

Based on all of the information you have gathered about your loved one, you have the opportunity to offer engaging activities that are appropriate and meet your loved one's personal preferences.

About the Authors

Scott Silknitter

Scott Silknitter is the founder of R.O.S. Therapy Systems. He designed and created the R.O.S. Play Therapy™ System, the *How Much Do You Know About* Series of themed activity books and the R.O.S. *BIG Book*. Starting with a simple backyard project to help his mother and father, Scott has dedicated his life to improving the quality of life for all seniors through meaningful education, entertainment, and activities.

Robert D. Brennan, RN, NHA, MS, CDP

Robert Brennan is a Registered Nurse and Nursing Home Administrator with over 35 years of experience in long-term care. He is a Certified Dementia Practitioner and is Credentialed in Montessori-Based Dementia Programming (MBDP) providing general and Train the Trainer programs. Robert was responsible for the development of an Assisted Living Federation of America (ALFA) "Best of the Best" award-winning program for care of individuals with dementia using MBDP. He currently provides education on dementia and long-term regulatory topics.

Dawn Worsley, ADC/MC/EDU, CDP

Dawn Worsley is a Certified Activity Director with a specialization in Education and Memory Care, a Certified Eden Alternative Associate, and a Certified Dementia Practitioner. With over 20 years of experience, Ms. Worsley is an authorized certification instructor with the National Certification Council of Dementia Practitioners and a Modular Education Program for Activity Professionals course instructor.

References

1. *The Handbook of Theories on Aging* (Bengtson, *et al.*, 2009)
2. *Activity Keeps Me Going, Volume 1,* (Peckham, *et al.*, 2011)
3. *Essentials for the Activity Professional in Long-Term Care* (Lanza, 1997)
4. *Abnormal Psychology*, Butcher
5. www.dhspecialservices.com
6. National Certification Council for Dementia Practitioners www.NCCDP.org
7. "Managing Difficult Dementia Behaviors: An A-B-C Approach" By Carrie Steckl
8. Iowa Geriatric Education Center website, Marianne Smith, PhD, ARNP, BC Assistant Professor University of Iowa College of Nursing
9. *Excerpts taken from "Behavior...Whose Problem is it?" Hommel, 2012
10. *Merriam-Webster's Dictionary*
11. "The Latent Kin Matrix' (Riley, 1983)
12. *Care Planning Cookbook* (Nolta, *et al.*, 2007)
13. "Long-Term Care" (Blasko, *et al.*, 2011)
14. "Success Oriented Programs for the Dementia Client" (Worsley, *et al.*, 2005)
15. Heerema, Esther. "Eight Reasons Why Meaningful Activities Are Important for People with Dementia." www.about.com
16. *Activities 101 for the Family Caregiver* (Appler-Worsley, Bradshaw, Silknitter)
17. American Foundation for the Blind
18. www.aging.com
19. www.WebMD.com
20. www.caregiver.org

RESOURCES:

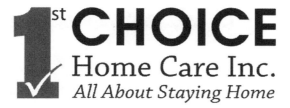

1st CHOICE
Home Care Inc.
All About Staying Home

1st Choice Home Care is **locally-owned** by Registered Nurses who have a working relationship with health care providers in the Triad. We are committed to providing **high quality** and **affordable** Home Care services to assist our clients to lead dignified and independent lives.

- ✓ Flexibility
- ✓ No contracts
- ✓ Personalized plan of care
- ✓ Compassionate and knowledgeable staff
- ✓ Access to a Registered Nurse at all times

Call us for a FREE in-home RN ASSESSMENT

336-285-9107

RESOURCES:

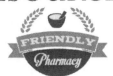

Modern Convenience, Old-Fashioned Service

3712-G Lawndale Drive
Greensboro, N.C. 27455

UBS FINANCIAL SERVICES

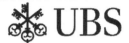

THE GREEN/DICKSON WEALTH MANAGEMENT GROUP

3200 Northline Avenue, Suite 100
Greensboro, N.C. 27408
(336) 854-7000

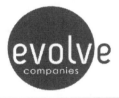

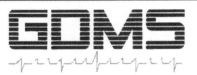

2310 Battleground Avenue
Greensboro, N.C. 27408
(336) 420-3943

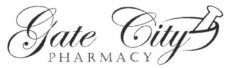

803 Friendly Center Road
Greensboro, N.C. 27408
(336) 292-6888

RESOURCES:

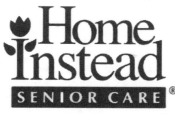

Home Instead
SENIOR CARE ®

To us, it's personal.

There really is "No Place Like Home". Home Instead Senior Care ® was created to help seniors remain safely in the comfort of their homes and to provide support to the family and friends who love them.

Since 1994, the Home Instead Senior Care network has been devoted to providing the highest-quality senior home care. That passion for quality has expanded our network to over 900 offices world-wide. Compassionate Home Instead CAREGivers[SM] are an invaluable resource in helping families eliminate worry, reduce stress, and reestablish personal freedom. All of our highly trained CAREGivers[SM] are bonded and insured for your peace of mind.

Since 2000, our Guilford County location has been providing premium services which are available around the clock and include services such as companionship, meal preparation, light housekeeping, medication reminders, respite care, and errands as well as continual, around the clock care and Alzheimer's care. Our experienced staff can help you find the right solution to assist your loved one in maintaining the best possible quality of life.

Home Instead Senior Care
4615 Dundas Drive, Suite 101
Greensboro, N.C. 27407
(336) 294-0081
www.HomeInstead.com/311

RESOURCES:

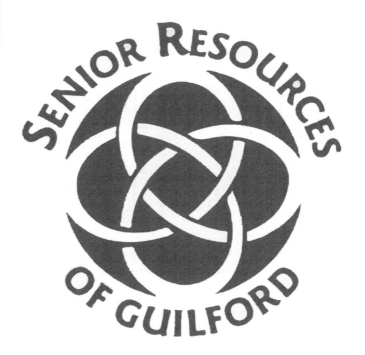

(336) 373-4816

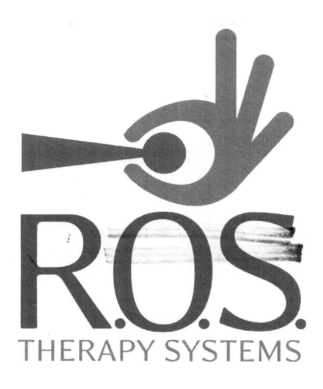

616.833 Silknitte 2015
Silknitter, Scott,
Activities for the family caregiver
30519010100553

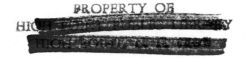

Made in the USA
Charleston, SC
20 October 2015